Lose Weight

The Top 100 Best Ways To Lose Weight Quickly And Healthily

By Ace McCloud

Copyright © 2014

Disclaimer

The information provided in this book is designed to provide helpful information on the subjects discussed. This book is not meant to be used, nor should it be used, to diagnose or treat any medical condition. For diagnosis or treatment of any medical problem, consult your own physician. The publisher and author are not responsible for any specific health or allergy needs that may require medical supervision and are not liable for any damages or negative consequences from any treatment, action, application or preparation, to any person reading or following the information in this book. Any references included are provided for informational purposes only. Readers should be aware that any websites or links listed in this book may change.

Table of Contents

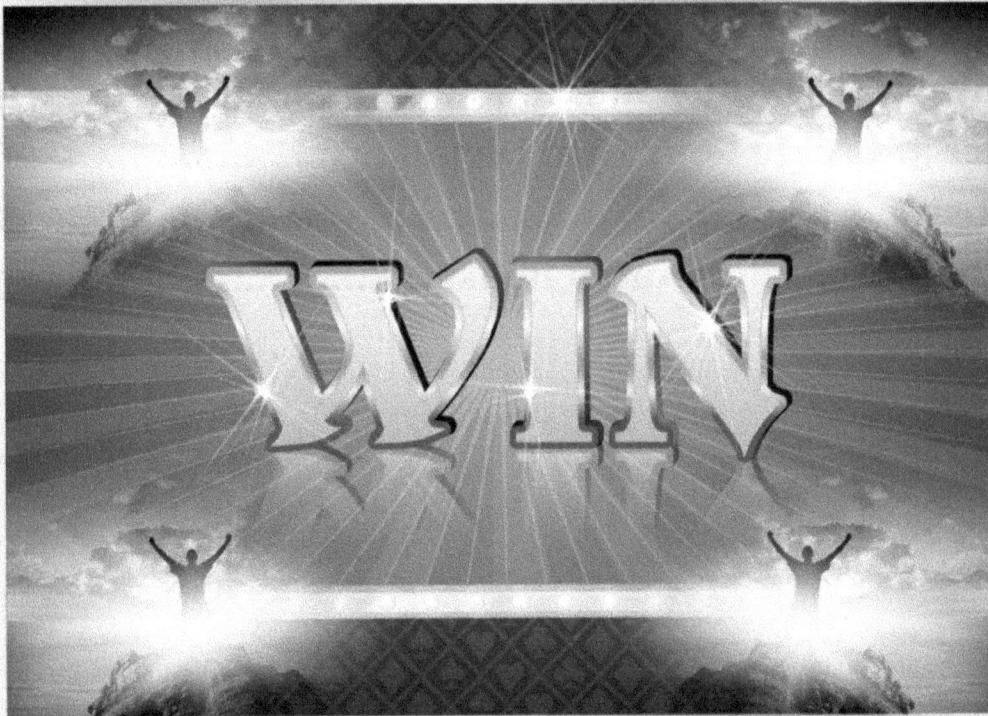

DEDICATED TO THOSE WHO ARE PLAYING THE GAME OF LIFE TO

WIN

KEEP ON PUSHING AND NEVER GIVE UP!

Ace McCloud

Be sure to check out my website for all my Books and Audio books.

www.AcesEbooks.com

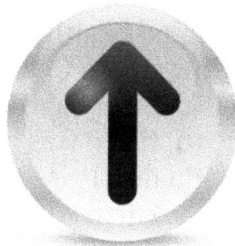

Introduction

I want to thank you and congratulate you for buying the book, "Lose Weight: The Top 100 Ways To Lose Weight Quickly and Healthily."

Weight loss is a hot topic in the United States and the world today. Between the desire to look great and the desire to be healthy, weight loss is often on the minds of many people every day. According to the Center for Disease Control, over one-third of American adults are considered overweight. That's almost 50% of the population! Between 1990 and 2010, there was a huge increase on average in the amount of weight put on by individuals. It is now an extremely serious topic as health systems are getting overwhelmed with obesity related sicknesses and problems. The goal of this book is to give you the best time tested methods for losing weight that are safe, effective, and healthy. Losing weight isn't as easy as looking in the mirror and saying, "Okay, I am going to lose 30 pounds!" Losing weight is a process that requires a good deal of time, focus, determination, and commitment. The good news is that it can be done very effectively with just a few changes to your daily routine.

When you're overweight, it is possible to face many unnecessary and negative health issues, such as type 2 diabetes, heart disease, strokes, physical injuries, and certain cancers. Many of these diseases and ailments can be fatal, but the good news is that many of them can also be prevented by staying within a weight that is healthy for your age and height. Also, not only can being overweight lead to many horrible medical problems, but it can also cost you—those who are considered overweight end up paying an average of $1,429 more on medical bills than those who are not.

If you are of non-Hispanic black descent, you are in the highest risk group for being overweight, followed by Hispanics, followed by Caucasians, followed by Asians. If you are a middle-aged adult, you are also in a higher risk group for becoming overweight. Interestingly, being overweight can be affected by certain socioeconomic factors as well. Women with college degrees are less likely to be overweight than women who do not have a high level of education, although the same does not apply to men. Black and Mexican-American men who are considered low-income tend to be less overweight than those with a higher income. Finally, women who earn a higher income are less likely to be overweight than women who earn a lower income. However, these are just statistics—anybody can be overweight, no matter what your race, ethnicity, income, or education level is.

Figuring out if you are overweight is simple. First, you can calculate your body mass index, or BMI. You can do this by dividing your weight by your height. The easiest way to figure it out is to let a BMI calculator do it—try it here. You can see exactly where you fall once you've punched in your weight and height. You can also figure out if you need to lose weight by measuring your waist or calculating your waist-to-hip ratio.

Take a minute and check out your BMI. Look on the right and see where you fall. Are you happy with the results? If not, read on, and learn about just how easy it is to lose weight and be healthy!

Being at a healthy and satisfying weight can help you increase your self-confidence and it can certainly help you live longer, as you may have a better chance at avoiding all the negative pitfalls that come with obesity. What is better than feeling strong, happy and healthy?

In this book, you'll learn 100 of the best ways to lose and maintain weight as well as how to design your own, customized diet and fitness plan to help you better manage your weight and lifestyle. Are you ready for a more energetic, fulfilling, and healthier life? Read on then and discover what you can do to shed those extra pounds!

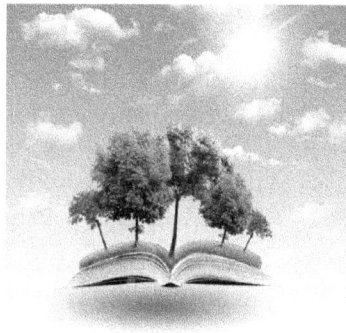

Chapter 1: The Modern Day Diet

The typical "modern-day" diet that the majority of people in the United States, England, and many others follow is not ideal for peak performance. In fact, many believe that it is actually contributing to the high rates of obesity.

There are several factors that influence the modern-day diet. First and foremost, the most common cause of weight gain is an imbalance in your energy. If you're not producing enough energy to match the amount of energy your body takes in, you pose a higher chance of being overweight. Putting "energy in" is basically whatever you eat and drink. Putting "energy out" is whatever actions your body takes throughout the day. This can be anything from simply breathing to performing high-intensity exercise. So, if you want to keep your weight stable, you need to balance your "energy in" and your "energy out." If you want to lose weight, you need to increase your "energy out." If you want to gain weight, you need to increase your "energy in."

The second most common cause of weight gain is having an inactive lifestyle. Many people are distracted by inactive activities, such as spending too much time in front of electronics, spending too much time at work, or spending too much time on school and homework. Another big factor toward weight gain is relying on modern technology instead of your own two legs for transportation. For example, instead of walking to work, you probably take your car straight there. Instead of taking the stairs to get somewhere in the mall, you may take the escalator.

The environment that you live in can also affect your weight. If you live in a place that does not have sidewalks, parks, or local gyms, it can be harder for you to stay in shape. Your work schedule can have negative implications on your ability to stay physical—many jobs have hours that are demanding, leaving some people with literally almost no extra free time to schedule in things like workouts. On that note, your income can have a direct impact on your health as well—healthier foods are often times more expensive than processed foods, and many of the best vitamins and nutritional supplements can be quite expensive as well.

If you're a person who works many hours, you may feel time constraints. You may not have a lot of time to cook or to go grocery shopping. This may lead you to become attracted to sugary snacks, which are often fast and popular on-the-go options. Many foods that are advertised to boost your energy are often filled with sugar, caffeine and empty calories, all of which are not great for your health. You may also be tempted to buy fast food or pre-packed, processed food, which many huge corporations have made as delicious and addictive as possible with more of a focus on profits than on the general wellbeing of their customers. If you think you are eating the right amount of food whenever you go out, you may be mistakenly be bringing in too much "energy." The Unites States, especially, is known for serving massive size meals. These huge meals are a major reason for weight gain. It is far better to have 4-5 smaller meals throughout the day than 2-3 big ones.

Finally, your family history and genes can sometimes dictate your weight. If your parents are overweight, your chances of becoming overweight can increase. Also, children tend to follow in the footsteps of their parents. So if your Mom or Dad is always eating unhealthily, your chances of doing the same are probably high too. Certain health conditions and medicines can also make you overweight, so it is important to always schedule an annual check-up with your doctor to help stay in tune with your health.

The factors that attribute to the modern day diet may seem overwhelming and intimidating, especially if you're so used to living your life the way you have been. Change can always seem like a scary thing. However, the good news is that any change to your "energy in" and "energy out" equation is often a positive change that can help you and your health for years to come. Later on in this book, you'll read about 100 easy and simple ways to help keep your weight off, many of which you can implement in your life no matter what your lifestyle is like.

Remember, the better health you are in, the easier it can be to maintain your weight and keep up high energy and mood levels. Here are some things to consider when it comes to taking care of your health:

Eating Right

Eating a healthy diet is one of the cornerstones of being able to maintain your weight. Ideally, your diet should follow the food pyramid, which suggests that you eat 6 to 11 servings of grains, bread, pasta, and cereal as well as 3 to 5 servings of dairy, 2 to 4 servings of fruit, and 2 to 3 servings of poultry per day, which rare use of fats, sweets, and oils.

Many magazines advertise fad diets that claim you can lose up to a certain amount of pounds in a certain amount of time, usually within a small time frame. Typically, they may help you lose weight in the short-term, but the weight will often come back due to unrealistic expectations and frustrations. Worse, you may even fall into discouragement and depression and end up gaining *more* weight than you started with.

However, following a realistic diet can help you lose and maintain weight. There are many great diets in existence, one of the most popular being the Mediterranean Diet. The Mediterranean Diet consists of a menu filled with food that people eat in the Mediterranean region. The diet and active lifestyle of those people has recently gained much attention since many Mediterranean people end up living into their 90's.

The Paleo Diet, another popular and effective diet, focuses on only eating all-natural, non-processed foods such as fresh vegetables and lean meat. The general idea is that for any diet to work, you will have to make a commitment to work hard and focus. A diet should really never last for just a short period of time. Instead, think of your diet as a lifestyle. The longer you can maintain your diet, the longer you can maintain your weight and overall health.

Exercise

Exercise is another cornerstone of maintaining a healthy weight and lifestyle. There are many different types of exercise. The most popular types of physical exercise include cardio and strength-training as well as the more advanced categories such as cross fit and high-intensity exercise. Mental exercise is important too. Great ways to practice mental exercises can be to try yoga or do some brain puzzles. Cardio exercises work out your lungs, which can help you boost your metabolism, fend off heart diseases, and better balance your hormones so that you will be less likely to feel depressed. Strength-training helps you build your muscles, which in turn builds confidence and helps burn fat. Yoga can help you build your muscles as well and it's a great method to help you clear your mind.

Supplements

When you eat a healthy diet, your body is more likely to receive the proper amounts of vitamins and minerals it needs to function. Vitamins and minerals are important for your body because they help your insides function properly. However, due to the many different types of diets (vegetarianism, vegan, Paleo, Mediterranean, etc) some people may not get enough of or the right amount of vitamins and minerals from the food they eat. Supplements can also be beneficial to you if you have any deficiencies, if you're pregnant, if you suffer from certain diseases, if you suffer from food allergies, or if you're just a really picky eater.

Before taking any supplements, you should always consult with your doctor, as your body may be different from another person who is reading this book. There is no "one size fits all" remedy when it comes to supplements. However, if your doctor has already given the okay for you to take supplements, it is important to be sure that you're taking the best ones possible. I personally have spent a minor fortune on supplements over the past twenty years, and it has been one of the best investments I have ever made. It takes a good amount of testing out and experimentation to find out what works best for you, but with a good strategy, you should be able to find some great items that help you function better both physically and mentally. For a more in-depth guide on supplements, exercises, and much more, be sure to check out my books: Ultimate Energy and Ultimate Health Secrets.

Chapter 2: The Top 100 Strategies for Losing Weight Quickly and Healthily

Now it is time to learn about some of the best ways to quickly and healthily lose weight. Before trying out any of these, please make sure that you've spoken to a health professional, as some of the strategies in this chapter may affect people differently.

Basic Habits:

Take It Slow. The first and most important strategy you should know about weight loss is to take small steps! Typically, people who lose weight end up gaining it right back within a few months. This is because your body can trigger a starvation alert, which can cause hormonal changes that bring you back to square one. This usually happens when people go for fad diets and "quick weight loss" schemes. While you *can* lose weight quickly, it is important to do it healthily and to work at in small amounts. This can help your body better adjust to metabolism changes. The more you focus on losing weight the right way, the more your hard work will pay off in the end!

Cleanse Your Body Before Starting. Although there is a wide debate about fasting and cleansing your body, some experts believe that it can be effective. The best strategy is to do this is once a year or right before you start trying to lose weight. A good cleanse can help reset your metabolism and help your taste buds to enjoy healthier foods.

Sleep Tight. Getting the right amount of sleep is a huge strategy that can help you keep the weight off. Your metabolism is at its strongest while you're sleeping, so the longer you sleep, the more calories you're able to burn off the next day. Without the proper amount of sleep, two hormones in your body can become unbalanced and cause you to have more cravings and feel less full. Not getting enough sleep can indirectly cause you to go for energy-boosting snacks that are filled with sugar, salt, and calories. Most adults should get around 8 hours of sleep each night, although older adults only need about 6.

Keep Your Commitment. Losing weight and keeping it off requires a lot of focus and strength. Although you can lose weight quickly and healthily, you will still need to keep your commitment fresh in your head if you want to keep it off. If you lose weight and then go back to your old ways, you will probably end up putting the pounds back on—that happens to a lot of people. Once you get into the habit of utilizing your new weight loss strategies, it can be much easier to keep your weight off. However, deciding to lose weight is a huge commitment, so before you start, you should try to clear up any relationship, personal, or work problems that you have in your life so you can fully concentrate on this. Also, be sure to let people know that you are trying to lose weight so that they can support you and hold you accountable.

What Motivates You? For quick and successful weight loss, you should have a main motivator. Everybody's motivation will be different, so you will need to sit back and think about yours. Do you want to look great at the beach this summer? Do you want to make sure that you're living healthily so you can watch your family grow? Before you get started, brainstorm a few of your motivations. Once you know what they are, you can be much more successful in reaching your goal of losing weight.

Have Support. When you're trying to do something by yourself, it can be hard to stay committed. If you're going to do something with a friend, your chances of going through with your commitment can be much higher. You and your friend can keep each other in check. Living healthily is a great goal, so you shouldn't have a hard time finding somebody to do it with. You could also meet other people with the same goal at the gym or at a weight loss support group.

Set Specific and Realistic Goals. Goal-setting is important because it can serve as the road map to your end result. Being specific is important because if you're too vague, you may not have a clear idea of how you're going to execute your goal. For example, if your overall goal is to lose 30 pounds, aim to lose at least 2 pounds each week and figure out what methods you'll try to do that. Don't try to lose 30 pounds in one week—that is unrealistic, and if you can't reach that Goal you may end up getting discouraged. It is also a good idea to start your goal off with the phrase: "I will easily..."

Know Your Metabolic Rate. Knowing your metabolic rate can help you figure out just exactly how many calories you should be eating per day. There are many free calculators online, such as this one, that you can use to plug in your specific figures. When you have this number, you can better plan your weight loss journey.

Exercise Habits:

Strength Training. The more your muscle mass you have, the more calories your body will be able to burn. Many people mistakenly pair strength training with aerobics, but to truly get your metabolism to where it will burn calories more rapidly, just stick to strength training in the beginning. You will learn more about some great strength training exercises in the next few paragraphs.

Do Squats. Squats are an easy exercise that you can perform almost anywhere to help keep weight off. To perform squats, stand with your feet aligned with the width of your shoulders and bend down so that your back is straight above the ground and your knees are parallel with your toes. To see this exercise in action, check out this YouTube video by POPSUGAR Fitness: How To Do A Squat Correctly.

Do Push-Ups. Push-ups are another great, easy, at home exercise that you can do anytime to help yourself lose weight. To do push-ups, get close to the ground and hold yourself up with your palms, positioned right under your shoulders. Bending your arms, slowly lower your body to the ground and then come up again. You can do push-ups in multiple reps for the best results. To see this exercise in action, check out this YouTube video on How To Do a Push-Up Correctly by Scott Malin.

Do a T-Push-Up. A T-Push-Up is a variation on the traditional push-up that works your abs a little better. To perform this exercise, do a regular push-up and then when you come back up, lift your hand and raise it over your shoulder as if you're making the letter T with your body. Bring your hand back down and do another push-up, this time raising your opposite arm. Repeat this exercise using multiple reps. To see this exercise in action, check out Passion4Profession's YouTube video on T-Push Ups.

Do Shoulder Press Push-Ups. Another type of push-up you an perform is a shoulder press push-up. To do this, you will need a bench of a chair. With your feet on your surface, put your hands on the floor, keeping them slightly more than shoulder-width apart. Lift your hips in the air, trying to stay as vertical as possible. Lowering your head to the floor, push yourself back to your starting position with your arms and shoulders. To see this exercise in action, check out this YouTube video: Perfect Pushup - Shoulder Press Pushup by Perfect Fitness.

Do Leaps or Skaters. To perform leaps, also known as skaters, position yourself as if you were going to squat but instead, put your weight on one foot and quickly leap to your other foot once you're halfway into the position. For the best results, do continuous reps of this exercise. To see this exercise in action, check out this YouTube video on How To Do a Leap/Skater by Howcast.

Try a Plank Crawl. This exercise can be a bit challenging but it is a great one to add to your list of weight loss exercises. To do a plank crawl, get on the ground and position yourself as if you were going to do a push-up. Slowly bend your forearms until you're in a planking position. Keeping your elbows right under your shoulders, push each arm up at a time until you're back into your original position. Try to do 15 to 20 of these per workout. To see this exercise in action, check out this Plank Crawl YouTube video by themoyermethod.

Do Some Walking Lunges. To perform a walking lunge, keep your arms at your side and stand with your feet apart. With your right foot, step forward, and bend your left knee 90 degrees. Keep your right knee parallel with your right ankle and don't let it go beyond your toes. To see this exercise in action, check out this YouTube video on How To Do a Walking Lunge by expertvillage.

Do Bird Dogs. Beginning on all fours, keeping your palms aligned with your shoulders and your knees aligned with your hips, extend one leg behind you and reach the same arm in front of you. Be sure to not arch your back and hold the position for a minute. You can slowly bring yourself back and repeat on the other side. To see this exercise in action, check out this YouTube video Bird Dog Core Exercise: 3 Variations by BuiltLean.

Perform a Bridge. To perform the bridge exercise, lay on your back, keeping your arms by your side. Keeping your feet flat on the floor, bend your knees and lift your body until your hips are aligned with your knees and shoulders. Hold this position for 3 seconds and repeat. To see this exercise in action, check out this exercise in action, check out this YouTube video on How To Do a Bridge by Howcast.

Do Pull-Ups. Like push-ups, pull ups are another great strength training exercise that can help you stay slim because they affect your body's biggest muscle. To properly perform a pull up, start by fully hanging with your hands shoulder-width apart. Then, pull yourself up until your chin goes over the bar and slowly lower yourself. To see this exercise in action, check out this YouTube video on the Perfect Pull Up - How To Do Pull Ups by Firm Butt Exercises.

Do Step-Ups. Step-ups are a great alternative to using a stair-climber and they do not require any special equipment. Using a step, quickly move your body up and down in a stepping motion. This can help you work your knee muscles and burn more calories. To see this exercise in action, check out this YouTube video on How To Do a Step-Up Correctly by Jerry Shreck.

Do Stick-Ups. Yes, there's another exercise with the suffix "ups" and it's called stick-ups. To perform this exercise, stand against a wall. Keep your feet half a foot from the wall. Hold your hands over your head, as if you're a part of a "stick up." Hold your elbows, shoulders, and wrists against the wall and tuck your elbows in, bring your arms down toward your sides. To see this exercise in action, check out this YouTube video on the Stick-Up Exercise by Cube Dweller Fitness.

Do V-Ups. A V-up is like a crunch except much more effective. To do a V-up, lie on your back and keep your legs straight. Holding your arms above your chest, contract your ab muscles and curl your body by lifting both your chest and upper legs. Keeping your back straight, stretch both end-points of your body together. Go back to your original position and repeat. To see this exercise in action, check out Athletic Muscle Building's YouTube video Abdominal Exercises - V-Ups.

Go Intense. During your workouts, don't let yourself rest for any longer than 30 seconds. This can seriously help your body to continuously burn calories.

Be Restless. Being restless and doing things such as repeatedly tapping your foot can actually benefit you. Tapping your feet, fidgeting, and other restless motions can help you burn up to 350 calories a day.

Spend Time in Nature. If you spend a lot of time in nature, chances are you could have a better chance at staying slim than others. Experts believe that is because people feel happier when they are outside. Many people prefer to walk outside than inside on a treadmill. Studies also show that walking outside can cut your cravings in half. Check out your local parks and see if there are any nice walking trails by your house.

Alternate Intensity. When exercising, kick it up a little every 20 seconds and then go back to your normal pace. This can help you take in more oxygen and you can burn fat faster.

Don't Get Lazy By Being Healthy. Have you ever put exercising off because you switched out a bag of chips for a plate of fruit? When you do something that is healthy, such as eating right, you pose a risk of putting off another healthy activity because you feel like you've already done something good. However, this trap can easily cause you to overeat, because you think you've already eaten light. Once again, be firm with yourself and get motivated to exercise anyway, even if you've already taken other positive steps toward weight loss. Just go ahead and start off with something easy, you may be surprised at how quickly you start to feel good and before you know it your work out will be complete.

Try Inline Skating. Inline skating can help you burn up to 425 calories within a half hour. This is because of the way your thigh and butt muscles move as you skate. For maximum results, skate strong and fast and then come to a medium pace for about thirty seconds to boost the amount of calories your body burns. Don't forget your protective gear!

Get Into Running. Running helps work your butt, leg, and core muscles, which are the main muscles that can help your body burn calories. In just a half hour, you can burn up to 374 calories. For the best results, run in a hilly area and keep your arms close to your body.

Invest in a Jump Rope. Jumping rope can burn as much as 340 calories in just a half hour. For the best results, keep your body upright and your feet apart and don't jump too high. If you don't have a jump rope, you can just jump.

Add a Hula Hoop to Your Workout. Hula hooping is a fun way to burn as much as 300 calories in a half hour. Hoops are inexpensive and easy to use. For maximum results, shift your weight back and forth between each foot. For even more fun, try to get some friends together and see who can go the longest.

Try Tennis. Tennis is a great way to burn up to 272 calories every half hour. It's a great workout because you have to use your arms to swing and you have to move back and forth and bend to pick up the balls. You can play with a friend or you can simply swing a ball against a flat wall.

Plug In and Dance. Dancing is a great and fun way to give your metabolism a jump-start. Although it can only burn up to 221 calories in a half hour, you can easily get lost in your favorite high tempo, upbeat songs. Really get into it. Wave your arms in the air and have some fun. One great idea is to make a playlist of your favorite workout songs.

Walk Vigorously. Don't forget about one of the simplest exercises—walking. Walking vigorously can burn as much as 170 calories in a half hour. However, the key is to be intense—taking a laid-back stroll won't do much. Take short, fast, and steady steps. For optimal results, walk for a while and then jog for a while, switching back and forth.

Take a Hike. Hiking can help exercise your core muscles. It's also a great way to spend time in nature. If you're feeling really ambitious, try mountain climbing! Both can help you build core muscles that can in turn help you burn fat.

Health Habits:

Watch Your Thyroid. One out of five adults who are over the age of 40 are at risk of suffering from an under-active thyroid, which can have negative effects on your metabolism. To keep an eye on your thyroid, it is important to schedule annual check-ups with your doctor. Some signs of having an under-active thyroid include fatigue, constant coldness, hair loss, poor circulation, and unexplained weight-gain that regular dieting cannot offset.

Drink Plenty of Water. Water can stop you from becoming dehydrated, which can then cause you to feel hungry when you're not. Water can help fill you up, so drink one glass of it before eating a meal. If you're concerned about the plain taste of water, you can substitute it for unsweetened green tea, which contains healthy, fat-burning antioxidants as an added bonus.

Get Enough Vitamin D. Vitamin D can help increase the effectiveness of leptin, which is a hormone that sends signals to your brain saying that you are full. Great foods to get vitamin D from include milk, yogurt, cheese, canned tuna in water, or sardines. Alternatively, you can use a vitamin D supplement.

Get Omega-3 Fatty Acid. Omega-3 fatty acids, which are commonly found in fish such as salmon, can help your body regulate your metabolism. Research shows that rats who took omega-3 supplements and then exercised lost more weight than rats that did not. If you're not a fan of fish, you could always get omega-3's by eating flaxseed oil, walnuts, or by taking an Omega 3 supplement.

Don't Starve Yourself. If you try to limit the amount of calories your body takes in, it could actually throw your metabolism off. Your body can actually stop burning fat in an attempt to save more energy. Be sure to eat—just be sure to make good eating decisions.

Practice Yoga. When you engage in yoga, you can lower the amount of stress in your life. The less stressed out you are, the less fat your body will absorb and store. Other relaxing, stress-killing activities include acupuncture and massages. These activities can help reduce inflammation, which can also fend off weight-gain. Massages can be costly so if you're willing to learn how to do it yourself, right in your own home, I highly recommend checking out my book The Best of Massage Therapy, Trigger Point Therapy, and Acupressure.

Know Your Body. If you begin to pay attention to how your body reacts after you eat, you can easily figure out when you're truly full, even if it means you didn't finish your entire plate. If you keep eating just because you have food leftover, you could eat up to an extra 500 calories a meal.

Laugh. You may have heard that laughter is great for combating stress but there is even better news—studies now show that laughing for just 15 minutes a day can increase your energy consumption by up to 40 calories! Learn how to make laughter a part of your day! For more information on learning how to live more lightly, please check out my bestseller: Laughter and Humor Therapy.

Anger and Resentment. Hatred, anger, resentment and other similar emotions are extremely detrimental to your overall physical and mental wellbeing. Being able to forgive the past and not keep dredging up unhelpful thoughts and memories can be very encouraging! For more information on exactly how to do this, you can check out my book on Forgiveness.

Eating Habits:

Eat Apples. Apples contain high amounts of pectin, which can help reduce the amount of fat your cells absorb. High in fiber, apples can help you stay full in between meals. For maximum results, eat an apple anywhere from an hour to a half hour before eating a meal.

Eat Oats. Since oats are in the category of whole grains, they are able to reduce your blood fat and cholesterol count. Like apples, oats can help you feel fuller. For the best results, try to incorporate oats into your breakfast. They are great as oatmeal and you can also make some pretty good shakes with them.

Eat Hulled Barley. One alternative to eating oatmeal for breakfast is to eat hulled barley instead. The latest research has found that hulled barley can stabilize your blood sugar, meaning you won't feel hungry later on. Be sure to stick to hulled barley and not processed barley, as the results may not be the same.

Sprinkle Cinnamon. Cinnamon does not have any calories and it can help you burn fat, making it an excellent spice to use. Cinnamon burns fat because it can help your body to better metabolize sugar. A great way to incorporate cinnamon into your diet is to add it your cereal, coffee, smoothies, or anything else you think it would go good with. You don't need a lot—just a up to 2 teaspoons at the most.

Eat Pine Nuts. Like apples and oats, pine nuts have the ability to make you feel fuller. They are also great for helping yourself resist cravings. If you're not a fan of pine nuts, you can substitute almonds for them. They basically have the same effects and are great for energy!

Eat Eggs. Despite the ideas that eggs are bad for you, they're actually quite good for quickly losing weight. The protein count in eggs can give you a huge burst of energy, especially in the morning. Studies have found that those who eat eggs in the morning as well as toast or cereal can lose twice the weight of those who eat a breakfast full of carbs.

Rethink Your Salads. Many people who are trying to quickly lose weight stick to eating plain salads with little to no dressing for lunch. However, this can leave you starving. By adding some fat and protein sources to your salad, you can stay full for much longer. Some ideas are to add chicken or light salad dressing to your salad to make it more exciting.

Replace Unhealthy "Quick" Snacks With Healthier Options. Instead of sinking a spoon into that tempting tub of ice cream or downing a quick candy bar, try to go for more healthier "to-go" options such as yogurt (which usually come prepackaged for easy travel), baked chips, raw vegetables, or fruit (apple slices are a popular option and also often come prepackaged for your convenience). Other healthy, fast snack options include individually packaged cheese sticks, mini whole-grain bagels with peanut butter and cinnamon, or hard-boiled eggs.

Get Minty. Mint is a very powerful substance. It can send signals to your brain that you're done eating and it can affect your taste buds in a way in which you won't want to load up on more food. After a meal, you can chew on some mint-flavored gum or suck on some peppermints. You can also use toothpaste that is minty. As an added bonus, brushing your teeth after each meal can also keep your oral health in the best shape.

Keep a Bottle of Hot Sauce Around. When you add hot sauce to your food, you will often eat slower and less of what's on your plate. Some experts even believe that the chilies used to make hot sauce can help to boost your metabolism. Keep a bottle of hot sauce handy and add it to any dish that it can go with.

Only Eat In Your Dining Room. In this day and age, it is common to eat almost everywhere *but* your dining room or kitchen. You may be used to eating in your car, in front of your TV, in front of your computer, or anywhere that is non-traditional. However, if you eat in your dining room or kitchen, you can reduce your chances of overeating. When you eat in places that you're more likely to snack in, you're more likely to eat more than you need.

Don't Forget Breakfast. There have been several debates as to whether it is beneficial or not to eat breakfast. However, if you eat a healthy breakfast, it can help you stay energized throughout the day, thus making you more likely to be on the go, which can help you burn calories. It can also help your body to adapt to new changes, such as metabolism shifts.

Eat Slowly. The slower you eat, the more full you'll feel. If you quickly gobble down your plate, you will find yourself still feeling hungry and wanting more. This technique is especially useful for eating dessert. Some people follow the rule of taking three bites and then letting go of their fork. Be sure to take small bites and savor each one. My younger brother has always had a weight problem, and one of the main contributing factors is that he would literally engulf his meals in almost no time. Take your time, enjoy your meal, and chew it up completely.

Start With a Protein Shake. If you prefer, you can switch out your breakfast with a protein shake. As long as it contains fortified nutrients, it can help you keep your weight off. Protein shakes are great for keeping you full and energized throughout the day. My favorite protein shake of all time is Muscle Milk.

No Midnight Snacks. Instead of treating yourself to a midnight snack, do not eat for at least two to three hours before you go to bed. Your metabolism changes and slows down as you sleep so instead of burning calories, you'd actually store them if you ate right before going to bed.

Question Cravings. We all get cravings, it's almost inevitable—especially when you're walking by a bakery and you smell the amazing odor of fresh bread, donuts, and cookies. However, if you're not really hungry and you're just craving something for the way it smells or looks, you will not be satisfied in the end and you may continue to eat. If anything, buy what you're craving and save it as a reward. Just remember the tip about midnight snacks.

Be Yourself in Social Situations. Have you ever gone out to eat with friends and indulged in dessert? Studies show that you tend to eat more when you dine with your friends. Women especially tend to go along with what others are doing, so if your friends are getting dessert or a second plate, chances are you will do the same. In situations like these, assert willpower and self-discipline. Tell your friends that you're comfortable with what you've had and you will just wait for them to finish.

Eat High Fiber Cereal for Lunch. Research shows that those who ate cereal instead of traditional meals ate 640 calories less than those who ate a typical diet. The best cereal choices are ones that are in high-fiber, served in low-fat milk.

Eat Dairy. Research shows that those who incorporate the standard amount of dairy into their diets were able to lose up to 11% of their body weight. Dairy can help your body break down fat better. Easy ways to get your dairy is to drink two 8-ounce glasses of milk, have a small cup of yogurt, and to eat an ounce of cheese.

Be Smart About Portion Control. Many people make the mistake of thinking that portion control is all about measuring food. While that is true, it is important to look at it in a different way, especially when you go out to eat. Restaurant meals tend to be oversized. You can always eat half and save the other half for later. You could also limit your intake of appetizers.

Cut Liquid Calories. Calories are abundant in food but you may forget to count the calories in your drinks. To keep your weight down, be sure to cut back on or avoid sugary drinks such as soda or fruit juice. Switch to water, flavored water, or unsweetened tea instead.   All three are healthy, delicious, and refreshing!

Aim for a Limited Diet. When you have many options to pick from, your chances of eating more can go up.   For example, one study showed that participants ate more fries when they were offered ketchup and mayonnaise to go with them. When you have more options to pick from, you tend to want to try them all. This is also true when you go out to eat at a buffet. To stick to this technique, exert some willpower and self-discipline. Tell yourself that you'll only stick to the healthiest of options. You'll soon notice that your willpower can pay off big time!

Eat More, Smaller Meals. If there is anything that I would like you to take from this book and actively use immediately, it is this! By eating more meals with smaller calorie counts, you can better resist cravings. It is also easier for your body to metabolize food, it is great for energy, and it is something that most of the peak performers and athletes around the world do! This is also a great strategy for eating fewer calories overall. Ideally you want to eat 4-5 healthy and smaller portioned meals throughout the day. I heard this advice many times when I was younger and never really listened to it. It wasn't until I finally started doing it that I was like "WOW"! This may be the number one tip to being healthy, energetic, and losing weight!

Avoid Trans Fats. Trans fats are bad enough for your body as it is but they are notorious for slowing down your metabolism.

Go Organic. You may have heard different things about organic foods but the truth is that organic foods are not sprayed with pesticides. Therefore, when you eat organic, your thyroid doesn't get exposed to toxins that could negatively impact your metabolism. Many grocery stores now offer organic foods at fair prices, so give it a try.

Buy Lean Meat. When grocery shopping, try to aim for meat that is 95% lean. Even 90% lean meat can still pack up to 10 grams of fat per serving. For chicken, breasts are the healthiest.

Eat Shrimp. Shrimp is a great food to buy for eating and snacking on because it has few calories, little fat, and lots of protein. You can easily buy ready-to-eat shrimp rings so you will not even have to do any preparing.

Eat Avocados. Research has found that eating half an avocado with your lunch can help curb your appetite. Women who did this reported feeling more satiated and had a decreased desire to snack in between meals.

Try Superfoods. Superfoods, such as beans, lentils, and chickpeas are loaded with healthy vitamins, minerals, and antioxidants. Research has also found that they can help you feel fuller and lessen your urge to snack in between meals. For more superfoods, be sure to check out my book: Ultimate Health Secrets.

Start With Low-Calorie Soup. Starting your meal with a small bowl of low-calorie soup is a great way to reduce the amount of calories you consume at once. Studies have found that those who ate soup before a meal were able to eat 20% fewer calories per meal.

Add Fermented Foods to Your Plate. Fermented foods, such as kimchi, pickles, or sauerkraut contain a fatty acid that can send appetite suppressing signals to your brain. They also contain a good type of bacteria that can help you digest food better.

Have a Cup of Coffee. While coffee should never be used as a substitute for energy, drinking one cup in the morning can help you boost your metabolism. This is because the caffeine in it can up your heart rate, therefore upping your metabolism about three hours after drinking it.

Snack on Dark Chocolate. Chocolate can be highly tempting even to those who have mastered the ability to exert willpower. If you are really craving chocolate, switch out milk chocolate for dark chocolate. Some experts believe that it can help you avoid cravings. One study found that those who ate dark chocolate before eating a meal ate 17% less calories.

Buy Frozen Vegetables. Vegetables are delicious and great for losing weight, but many people are turned off from having to prepare them—washing them, slicing them, etc. To avoid this, just stock up on some bags of frozen vegetables. They're cost-effective, you can store them for longer, and most of them can be cooked right in the microwave and come out tasting fresh.

Store Healthy Food at Eye Level. Instead of keeping unhealthy food close by; keep your healthy snacks on hand. Store them in the fridge right where you can see them or in the most obvious place in your pantry. You'll likely go for the healthier option if it's right in front of you.

Chill Out. Other research has found that spending time in places that are between 55 and 65 degrees Fahrenheit can help your "good" fat rev up your metabolism so that it burns more calories. While this may not make a huge difference overnight, it can certainly help you. Just be sure not to eat more if you get too cold.

Don't Keep Unhealthy Snacks in the House But Go Out For Them. Amidst your weight-loss journey, you should definitely cut back on how many treats you consume but you certainly shouldn't torture yourself either. It is okay to treat yourself to an unhealthy snack once in a while. The key is to go out for them. If you love chocolate ice cream, don't keep it in the house, where you're more likely to have access to it—instead, go out to the ice cream shop. You will only get as much as you buy, so you won't eat too much of it.

Snack on Greek Yogurt. Greek yogurt is a great snack you can have to help yourself lose weight because it is packed with fiber and protein. It also contains plenty of Vitamin C, which can help boost your metabolism. For a really great snack, try adding raspberries and honey to it.

Snack on Grapes and Walnuts. A small cup of grapes and walnuts is a great snack because they contain plenty of fiber, natural sugars, and protein, all of which can make you full and become more energized. The more energetic you are, the more likely you will be motivated to move around and burn more calories.

Snack on Edamame. Edamame is a great snack because it's packed with fiber and protein. Moreover, research has shown that you're more likely to feel filled if you can see the remains of your food. Edamame comes in pods, which you often leave behind after sucking the insides out.

Snack on Wheat Crackers and Cottage Cheese. This snack can help you stay full in between meals, especially if you choose regular cottage cheese for the low-fat option—the fat in the regular kind contains more protein to help you stay more full.

Snack on Hummus with Cucumbers and Olives. This snack is a Mediterranean style snack, derived from the Mediterranean diet. Each component is low in fat and high in fiber. They also all go really well together.

Snack on Bananas with Peanut Butter. The carbs and the protein that you can get out of this snack can help you stay energetic and in a good mood, which can help you keep going all day.

Snack on Pear Slices and Almond Butter. Putting together slices of pears with almond butter on top can be a great carb and protein combination. You can also add some cinnamon on top, making it extra healthy.

Don't Get Whipped Cream. If you're a coffee-lover, especially the dessert-type coffees, try to say no to the extra whipped cream that often comes on top of them. By skipping the whipped cream, you can lower the calories dramatically. If you're really in the mood for whipped dream, get it on an espresso shot, which only has around 30 calories.

Be Smart About Dessert Drinks. Cocktails and other dessert drinks can often contain huge amounts of calories due to the syrups, sugars, and other additives that go into them. To have a healthy drink after dinner, stick to ones that contain tonic water, club soda, cranberry juice, or citrus.

Motivation Habits:

Have "Weight-Loss" Jeans. To really help yourself stay motivated, you can find a pair of jeans that are tight-fitting on you. Make sure you can zip them up. Try them on before every weekend, when you're more likely to splurge. If you can start fitting into them comfortably, you'll be more likely to stick to your new lifestyle.

Weigh Yourself Frequently. Many people believe that weighing themselves frequently is a sign of an unhealthy weight-loss obsession, but it can actually help you keep track of where you are. If you start to gain weight again, you can catch it early and rethink your strategy and lifestyle. If you wait too long to weigh yourself, you may find that all of your hard work went down the drain and you may be discouraged to try again.

Start in May. If your timing is right, start your weight-loss journey in May. Starting in May is effective because the days last longer and your energy will still be full by dusk. It stays light out longer so you can always squeeze in extra outdoor exercise after work.

Make It A Competition. If you're a competitive person or if you're looking for a way to make weight-loss more fun, get a friend to do it with you and see who can reach their goals first. This can motivate you to keep your focus and dedicate more time to losing weight. It's an easy and fun way to get into the habit of living healthily.

Take Photos. One great way to stay motivated toward losing weight is to take before and after pictures. Any time you're feeling tempted to give up, take out those pictures and look at them. Compare them to yourself now. More often than not, you'll probably be more inspired to stick to being healthy.

For more information on getting yourself motivated, be sure to check out my books on: Motivation and Inspiration.

Cooking Habits:

Measure Your Cooking Oil. Many recipes call for cooking oil but some oils can have up to 120 calories in each tablespoon. Many recipes don't even tell you how much to use—it just calls for a thin coat. You may often mistake that for filling your pan with too much oil. To reduce the amount of calories you get from oil, put enough in to just thinly cover the surface of the pan. If you're using a non-stick pan, you will not need to use much oil at all. Also, whenever possible, use Coconut Oil. Coconut Oil has been found to be extremely healthy in a variety of different ways.

Measure Ingredients Accurately. If you try to guess how much is enough of certain ingredients, you may end up cooking too much of something, which can lead to overeating. For example, you may try to guess what one pound of meat looks like, but unless you have a scale, you might not know for sure.

Have a Healthy Snack Before You Cook. If you cook on an empty stomach, chances are that you can accidentally overeat by "tasting" your creation as you go along. Then, when you sit down to actually eat it, you may not count the amount of food that you tasted. To avoid this, you should eat a light, healthy snack before you get ready to cook.

Don't Follow Recipes Exactly. Following recipes is important for having a meal turn out good, but you don't always have to follow it exactly. For example, if the recipe calls for white bread, substitute it with two slices of whole grain bread. Making simple switches like this can easily help you stay slim.

Only Make as Much Food as You Need. Pay attention to serving size when you begin to make your own meals. Some recipes can lead you to make enough food for 10 people. When you have more food than you really need, your chances of overeating can go up. To avoid this, you can tweak the recipe so that you only make enough for yourself or you can freeze the rest of the food for later.

Use Small Plates. The bigger your plates are, the more likely you are to fill them up and overeat. Instead of using standard-sized dinner plates, try to stick with half-size plates. Keep your dinner plates for salads, which are okay to eat in bigger portions.

Juicing and Smoothies. Juicing and smoothies are absolutely incredible for great health, energy, losing weight and maintaining an ideal body weight. I can't recommend both of them enough! I have also noticed a great boost in energy levels after juicing, especially if done on a regular basis. Smoothies are incredible as well, and great for a quick morning meal or an afternoon snack. A great juicer is the Breville Juice Fountain and I highly recommend the Nutri-Bullet Smoothie

Blender. If you haven't gotten into smoothies or juicing, it is something that you should definitely check out.

Chapter 3: Create Your Own Diet Plan

Making your own customized diet plan is a great way to get started on your weight loss journey. When you design your own plan, your chances of sticking to it can be much higher because it will be fresh in your head and controlled by you. All you need to get started is a blank notebook and some great ideas, which you can read about in this chapter! Since creating your own diet plan can seem overwhelming at a glance, I will take you through it step-by-step so that you can confidently move forward.

Step One

One of the most important components of a diet plan is figuring out how many calories you should eat each day. To figure this out, you will need to use another calculator that can take your information and come up with a number for you. Freedieting.com has a really good one, which you can access here. I like this calculator because it tells you how many calories you need to maintain your weight and how many you need to lose it.

Once you have a better idea of what your average daily calorie intake should be, the next step is to become more familiar with the major food groups. Since your diet plan is totally up to you, the simplest way to design your plan is to map it out by using units of food. So, for example, you'll be organizing each meal by food type—fruits, vegetables, proteins, whole grains, leafy greens, and protein. By doing this, you can make it much easier to remember what you're going to eat for every meal.

So, for example, if you were going to create a diet plan based on 1,500 calories per day, it may look something like this:

Breakfast: One protein source and one fruit source

Lunch: One protein source, one vegetable source, unlimited leafy greens, one whole grain source, and one fruit source

Snack: One protein source and one vegetable source

Dinner: Two protein sources, one whole grain source, two vegetable sources, and unlimited leafy greens

Do you now see how you can take this and sort of "fill in the blanks?" Let's give it a try:

Breakfast: Half a melon, filled with regular cottage cheese; one glass of skim milk

Lunch: One cup of low-fat yogurt with apple slices; brown rice with vegetable of your choice (maybe onions and carrots); and an optional leafy green of your choice

Snack: One hard-boiled egg and a handful of mini peppers (preferably red peppers, remember what spicy food can do for you as you learned in Chapter 2?)

Dinner: Salmon with parsley and red-wine sauce; steamed broccoli; and brown rice with vegetables mixed in

Remember, this is just an example of how you can fill-in-the-blanks of your diet plan! Review Chapter 2 and see what kind of muscle-building, fat-burning foods you can incorporate into your own plan. One of the best parts about creating your own diet plan is that it never gets boring. You can always switch it up and experiment when you get tired of eating the same dishes over and over again!

Step Two

Now that you have a good idea on how to arrange your diet plan, I have some breaking news—it's not over yet and it's not *that* easy (although it is generally very easy if you do things right! Don't get discouraged! Next, you have to know a little bit about portion size and control, or else your plan may not work at all. Without knowing how to manage your portions, you could end up overeating or going over your calorie count without even knowing it!

Since you now know how to organize your diet plan based on units of food, I will give you some insight on how to quickly and easily measure your portions based on those units. Many products that you buy in the store will tell you the nutritional value and serving size right on the label. For now, however, I will give you a general overview of the most common portions for each unit:

For protein, one unit is equivalent to 250 grams (or 1 cup) of non-fat cottage cheese or yogurt. Either one can be plain or vanilla-flavored. One unit of protein is also equal to 3 ounces of cooked lean meat or chicken, 4 ounces of cooked fish, or one egg.

One unit of fruit is equivalent to a palm-sized amount of dried fruit, 125mL (or half of a cup) of 100% fruit juice (be wary of fruit juices that secretly contain sugar), 80 grams (or one cup) of sliced fruit, or one whole fruit, such as a whole apple or orange.

For vegetables, 80g (or 1 cup) of any vegetable counts as one unit. You can eat as many leafy greens as you want.

One unit of a grain is equivalent to any half cup of rice, beans, pasta, peas, or corn. A slice of whole grain bread also counts. Additionally you could substitute a half of a white or sweet potato, or 250 grams (1 cup) of rolled oats.

When it comes to having a snack, just be smart. Obviously, a bag of chips or a candy bar will not help you lose weight. Instead, go for something like an organic protein bar, a glass of skim milk, a few tablespoons of hummus, a low-fat cheese stick, almonds, or a small cup of soybeans.

Finally, don't let your diet plan make you lose your taste for food! There are many great, healthy taste enhancers you can add to your food so that it stays exciting and delicious. For cooking your meals, I highly recommend cooking with extra virgin olive oil or coconut oil, those two oils are the best kind for your health. If you're having a salad, make it more "fun" by adding a couple of tablespoons of low-fat dressing, avocado, grated cheese, or nuts. You can still indulge in your favorite condiments, such as ketchup or mayonnaise (preferably low-fat), just be sure to be aware of how much you're using!

Step 3: Make a Menu

Step 3 will probably be the most fun! Make it a goal to create a menu for yourself at the beginning of every week. Planning your meals out in advance can help you save time and money during the week. When you come home from work every night, you'll already know what you're having and when you're at the grocery store, you'll know exactly what you need to buy for the week. You don't have to physically create a menu but you should at least have a good idea in your head of what your week is going to look like in terms of eating.

Here is a good example of a menu that you could use for yourself for one week:

Monday

Breakfast: Oatmeal with blackberries and a glass of skim milk

Lunch: Spinach salad with grilled chicken, light dressing, nuts, and shredded cheese and a cup of green tea

Snack: Apple slices with peanut butter

Dinner: Grilled salmon with brown rice, broccoli, and mashed potatoes and iced green tea

Tuesday

Breakfast: Two slices of whole-grain toast with all natural peanut butter, banana slices, and sprinkled cinnamon and a glass of fresh orange juice

Lunch: Grilled chicken panini on a whole wheat roll with black forest ham and Swiss cheese and a glass of water

Snack: Handful of dried berries

Dinner: Roman Chicken with whole wheat pasta, steamed vegetables, and a cup of tea

Wednesday

Breakfast: Strawberry oatmeal smoothie

Lunch: Mozzarella and Tomato salad with iced green tea

Snack: One cup of flavored Greek yogurt

Dinner: Turkey burgers, sweet potatoes, a garden salad, and a glass of water

Thursday

Breakfast: Two hard-boiled eggs and a glass of juice

Lunch: Chicken quesadillas with goat cheese and a glass of water

Snack: Cup of sliced veggies with light ranch dip

Dinner: Grilled steak topped with mushrooms, tomatoes, and green beans and a glass of water

Friday

Breakfast: Scrambled eggs and whole wheat toast with a glass of skim milk

Lunch: Cucumber and turkey sandwich with garlic and horseradish and a glass of water

Snack: Mozzarella cheese stick

Dinner: Zucchini flat-bread sandwich with hummus, goat cheese, and Arugula with a cup of tea.

So, just by looking at that sample menu, you can plan on buying plenty of vegetables at the grocery store as well as chicken, steak, a dozen eggs, lots of green tea bags, juice, oatmeal, dried fruit, and small healthy snacks. By knowing what ingredients you'll need for the week, you can more easily pass over the junk food aisles or on buying foods that you really don't need.

Step 4: Make a Fitness Plan

Do you remember when I talked about how important exercising is for losing and maintaining weight? Don't forget to work out a fitness plan along with your menu as part of your custom diet plan. There are many ways to customize your own fitness plan, depending on your lifestyle and schedule. Let's take a look at a few different scenarios so you can have an idea of what your fitness plan will look like:

For Somebody With Kids: Instead of handing the kids off to a babysitter and hitting the gym, schedule in a nice, long walk in the park or around your neighborhood. Kids will probably be into playing a fun sport, like basketball or soccer. Both sports are a great way to get in some cardiovascular activity. Getting kids involved with exercise as early as possible is a great way to help them get into the habit of taking care of their bodies. It can also make exercising very fun.

For Somebody Who Works Crazy Hours: Instead of giving up on exercise altogether, be smart about what you do. Park your car a few blocks away from your office and enjoy a nice walk to and from work every day. You could also buy a small set of portable weights and keep them in your office so that you can use them whenever you have free time. Another option is to get up an hour or two early and take a jog or hit a gym for more intense exercise.

For Somebody With a Home Gym or Gym Membership: If you have access to a home gym or gym membership with a fairly decent schedule, try to get in 30-50 minutes of cardio exercise three to five times per week and plan on doing strength exercises twice a week. Strength training works your core muscles so it is essential to allow them to rest. Here is a sample schedule:

Monday: 30 minutes of kickboxing

Tuesday: 30 minutes of vigorous walking and a strength training set

Wednesday: 30 minutes of playing basketball

Thursday: 30 minutes of swimming or jogging and a strength-training set

Friday: 30 minutes of cycling

Note: If you are a beginner or not in the greatest shape, or just want a great work out with little risk of injury, then just walking is perfectly fine. It is a great work out, low impact, easy to do and maintain, and has incredible benefits. Walking and swimming are my two favorite forms of cardio exercise.

Step 5: Make a Commitment

The final step in creating your own diet plan is to make a commitment to yourself that you will stick to it. Creating it can be simple but actually following it can be a little more challenging.   To help you stay inspired to follow your plan, pick a few role models who have also lost weight in a safe and healthy manner and strive to do the same. If you're having trouble becoming motivated to stick to your plan, take advantage of the "power of why." Why do you want to lose weight? Maybe it's because you want to look great for the summer, meet new people, protect yourself against certain diseases, have more energy, live longer, or have a better sex life.   Staying inspired and motivated can dramatically help you exert willpower and self-discipline. For more information on mastering any of these skills, I invite you to check out my other bestselling books: Inspiration and Influence, Willpower, and Self-Discipline.

Conclusion

I hope this book was able to help you to get a better idea of where you are in terms of your weight and losing it. Moreover, I hope you were able to learn about some of the best and easiest ways to reach your desired end result!

The next step is to get started. First, take a picture of yourself as soon as you can after reading this book. That will serve as your "before" photo, your inspiration. Download it to your computer, print it out, share it on social media, or do whatever it takes to remind yourself that you want to change your life. Next, go back to Chapter 2 and pick something from each category to start trying. Once you've mastered those few things, go back and pick a few more from each section to implement into your life. It will take some time and definitely a lot of focus, but if you can push yourself to get into these healthier habits, you can start losing weight in almost no time! Don't forget to start experimenting with your diet and fitness to find out what works best for you! Once you have found out what is giving you the best results, make them into a Habit! Be sure you have your goals firmly in place and somewhere that you can read them often. Lastly, don't forget to take an "after" photo and share it with your supporters once you've succeeded!

Finally, if you discovered at least one thing that has helped you or that you think would be beneficial to someone else, be sure to take a few seconds to easily post a quick positive review. As an author, your positive feedback is desperately needed. Your highly valuable five star reviews are like a river of golden joy flowing through a sunny forest of mighty trees and beautiful flowers! *To do your good deed in making the world a better place by helping others with your valuable insight, just leave a nice review.*

Thanks and Best of Luck

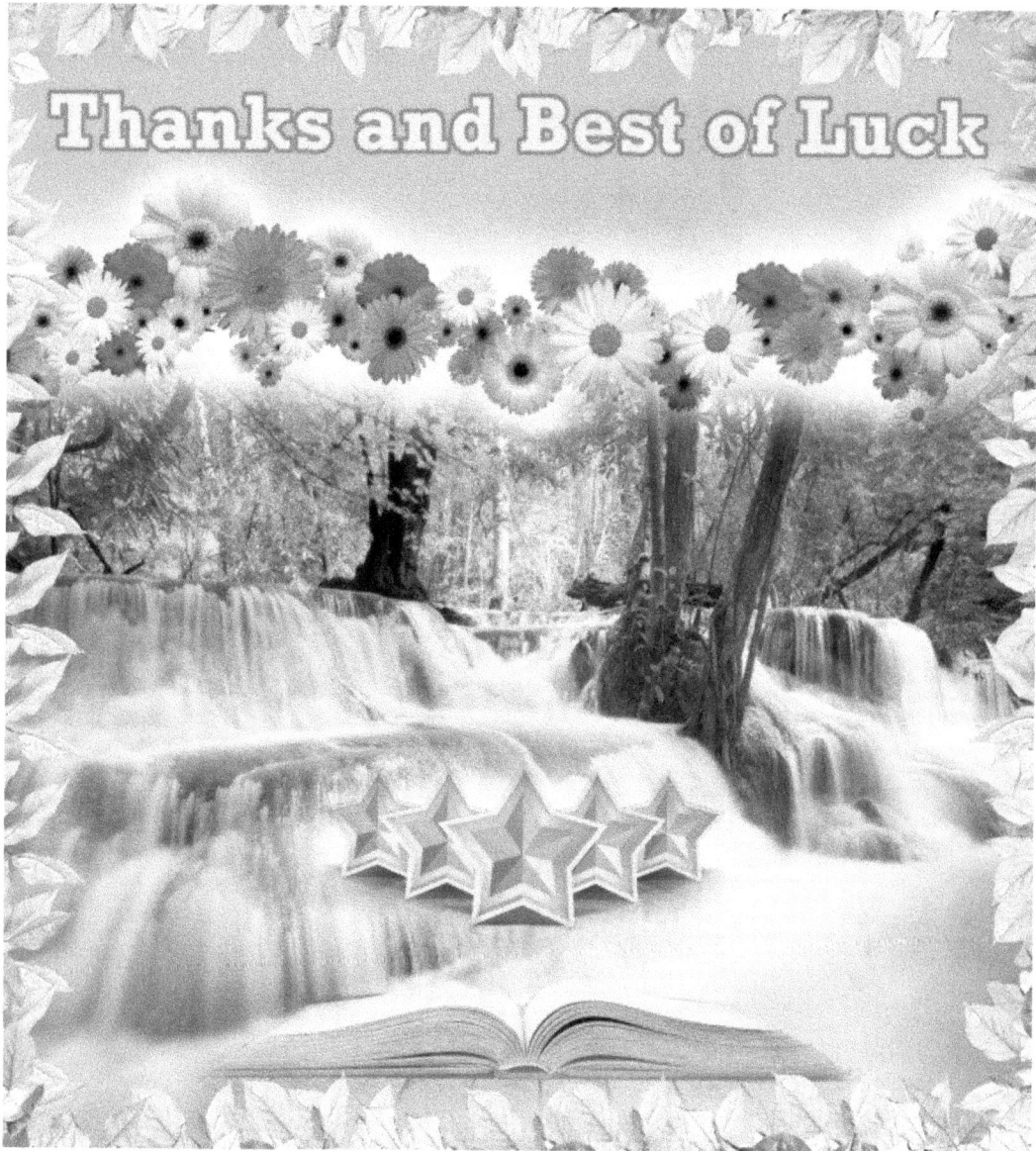

My Other Books and Audio Books
www.AcesEbooks.com

Health Books

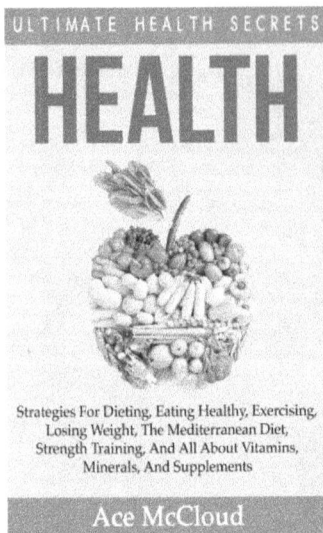

ULTIMATE HEALTH SECRETS

HEALTH

Strategies For Dieting, Eating Healthy, Exercising,
Losing Weight, The Mediterranean Diet,
Strength Training, And All About Vitamins,
Minerals, And Supplements

Ace McCloud

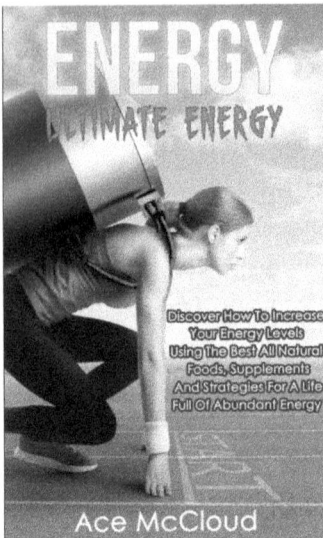

ENERGY
ULTIMATE ENERGY

Discover How To Increase
Your Energy Levels
Using The Best All Natural
Foods, Supplements
And Strategies For A Life
Full Of Abundant Energy

Ace McCloud

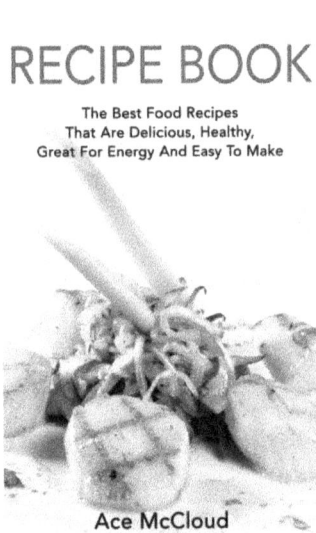

RECIPE BOOK

The Best Food Recipes
That Are Delicious, Healthy,
Great For Energy And Easy To Make

Ace McCloud

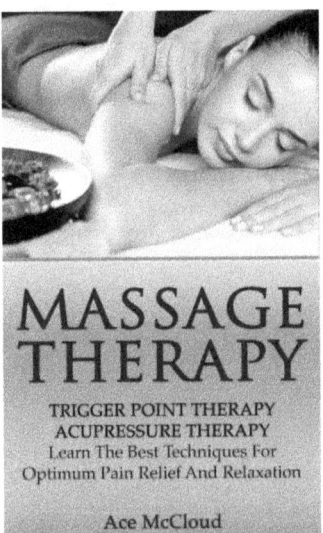

MASSAGE THERAPY

TRIGGER POINT THERAPY
ACUPRESSURE THERAPY
Learn The Best Techniques For
Optimum Pain Relief And Relaxation

Ace McCloud

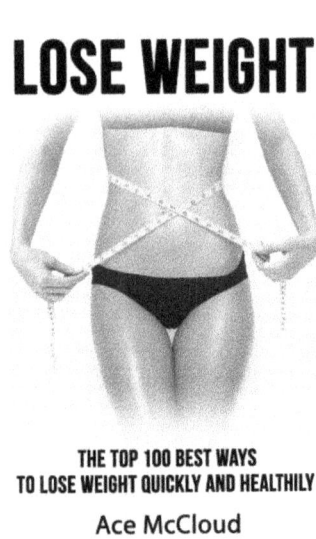

LOSE WEIGHT

THE TOP 100 BEST WAYS
TO LOSE WEIGHT QUICKLY AND HEALTHILY

Ace McCloud

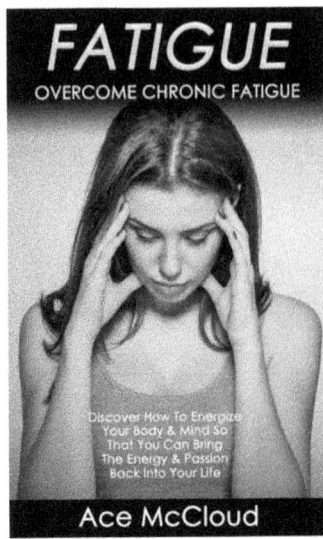

FATIGUE
OVERCOME CHRONIC FATIGUE

Discover How To Energize
Your Body & Mind So
That You Can Bring
The Energy & Passion
Back Into Your Life

Ace McCloud

Peak Performance Books

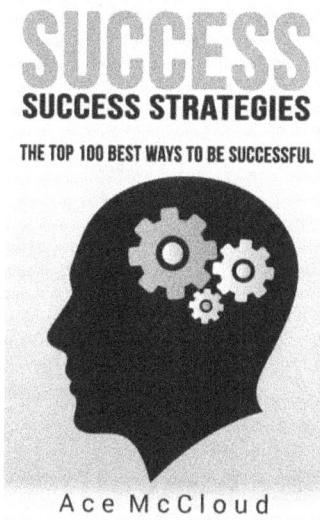

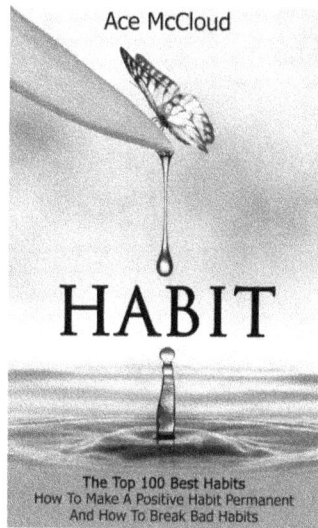

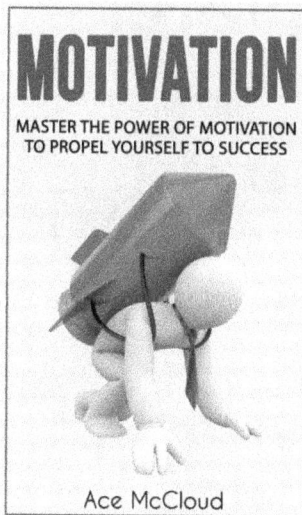

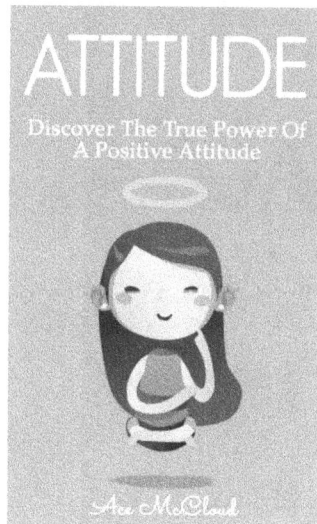

SUCCESS
SUCCESS STRATEGIES
THE TOP 100 BEST WAYS TO BE SUCCESSFUL

Ace McCloud

Ace McCloud

HABIT

The Top 100 Best Habits
How To Make A Positive Habit Permanent
And How To Break Bad Habits

MOTIVATION
MASTER THE POWER OF MOTIVATION
TO PROPEL YOURSELF TO SUCCESS

Ace McCloud

ATTITUDE
Discover The True Power Of
A Positive Attitude

Ace McCloud

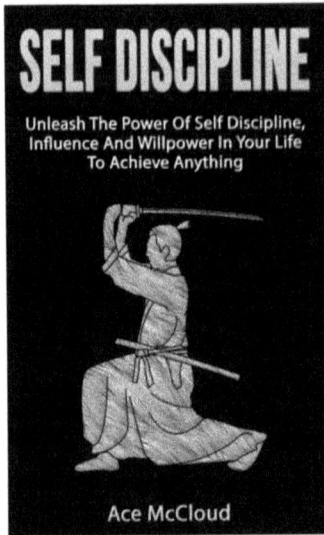

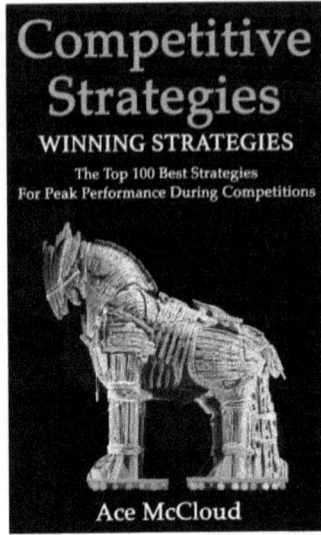

Be sure to check out my audio books as well!

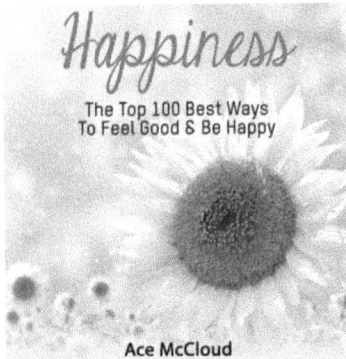

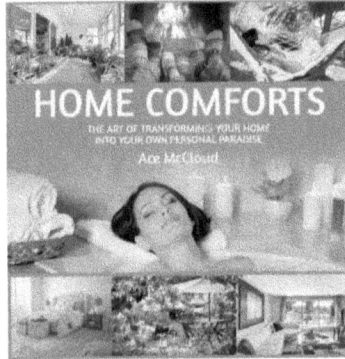

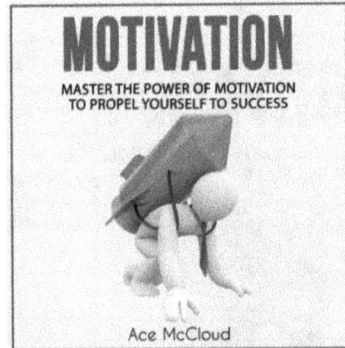

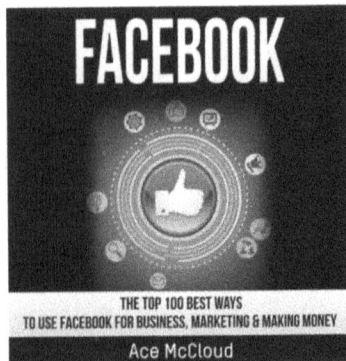

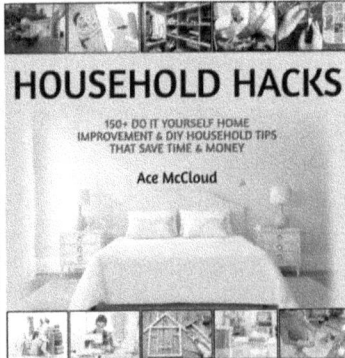

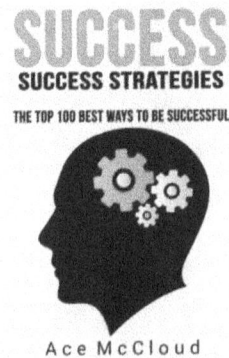

Check out my website at: **www.AcesEbooks.com** for a complete list of all of my books and high quality audio books. I enjoy bringing you the best knowledge in the world and wish you the best in using this information to make your journey through life better and more enjoyable! **Best of luck to you!**

www.ingramcontent.com/pod-product-compliance
Lightning Source LLC
Chambersburg PA
CBHW080632030426
42336CB00018B/3168